Table of Contents

Alcohol and Brain Aneurysms: Risk Factors, Symptoms, and More

1. Introduction to Brain Aneurysms and Alcohol Consumption

It is possible to lower your risk of experiencing a brain aneurysm by eating healthily and staying active. In fact, abstaining from or consuming alcohol for 7-13 units weekly could account for a 7% reduced risk of brain aneurysms. Drinking more alcohol, however, could increase your risk. According to medical research, consumption of 14-24 units of alcohol per week can increase the likelihood by 8%, and 25 units or more by 16%. It is important to understand how substances like alcohol could impact a patient's risk of developing a brain aneurysm and the possibility of it rupturing.

A brain aneurysm is a bulging, weak area in the wall of an artery in the brain, which can burst and cause a hemorrhagic stroke if it leaks. According to medical research, certain lifestyle factors such as becoming dehydrated, high blood pressure, and becoming overly excited – which can be induced through laughter or even heavy exercise – can all trigger a brain aneurysm to leak or burst. If an aneurysm has ruptured, you may not experience symptoms. However, the most common sign is severe headaches that are sudden and accompanied by vomiting and a stiff neck.

2. Understanding Brain Aneurysms

There are two types of brain aneurysms: unruptured and ruptured. A "giant" aneurysm is an abnormally large aneurysm, and a "fusiform" aneurysm lacks the natural neck that regular aneurysms have and involves a dilation of the entire circumference of the artery. Both may have a higher risk of rupture. In the general population that experiences headaches, aneurysm is still an uncommon cause of a headache: nonaneurysmal SAH, primary thunderclap headache, and cervical artery dissection were found to be responsible for headaches 70% of the time, and "warning headaches" were found to be associated in about 19% of people between ages 25 and 75 who have an unruptured brain aneurysm (neither rate may be higher per individual clinical situation). The prevalence of aneurysms varies by different populations and risk. The annual incidence of aneurysms in different countries based on autopsies has been estimated at 0.4% to 10.5%, and the annual incidence of subarachnoid hemorrhage is estimated to be 0.7 to 12.8 per every 100,000 people.

An aneurysm is a bulge or ballooning in an artery in the body. These bulging areas tend to form where the artery wall is weak or has become weakened over time. In the brain, an aneurysm can cause a hemorrhagic stroke that occurs when blood escapes into the space around the brain or into the brain tissue itself. This can damage brain cells in one of two ways: Intracerebral hemorrhage occurs when an aneurysm in the brain ruptures and bleeds into the tissue of the brain near the aneurysm. Subarachnoid hemorrhage occurs when an aneurysm ruptures and bleeds into the space between the brain and the skull (the subarachnoid space). About 30,000 cases of subarachnoid hemorrhage due to a ruptured cerebral aneurysm occur in the U.S. each year. This type of hemorrhage can lead to brain damage, heart attack, or death.

2.1. Definition and Types of Brain Aneurysms

A brain aneurysm is considered a brain disease due to the brain's blood vessels covering the entire brain, and arteries can be found anywhere on the surface of the brain. Aneurysms, especially berry aneurysms, which are usually found at the base of the brain, are sometimes impossible to operate on. When they are treated, the consequences can be very severe sometimes. Symptoms that are caused by having a brain aneurysm can include weakness, headache, hearing sounds unheard by others, seeing colors, etc. Brain aneurysms can cause bleeding in the brain as well. If a brain aneurysm soon causes symptoms, this generally means that the aneurysm has ruptured (burst). If an unruptured brain aneurysm becomes symptomatic, it usually presents with a debilitating headache, similar to a sentinel headache. However, rupture is associated with significant morbidity and mortality, which is why it is important to identify unruptured aneurysms before they rupture. In some cases, a computerized tomogram of the head, magnetic resonance angiography, or catheter angiogram is essential to identify a brain aneurysm.

Aneurysms can happen to anyone, as all ages of people run a risk. However, factors that can increase the risk of having brain aneurysms are: family history of brain aneurysms at an early age, United States Japanese descent, and aged between 40-55 years. Drug abuse, polycythemia, alcoholism, and many other factors can also increase the risk of brain aneurysms.

1. A berry aneurysm is a saccular aneurysm, the most common type of brain aneurysm, and is usually found at the base of the brain. 2. A berry aneurysm got its name because it looks like a small berry hanging from a tree.

A brain aneurysm is a bulge in the wall of one of the arteries of the brain. These are generally weak or thin and balloon out to form a pocket. There are two most common types of brain aneurysms: sacculated and berry aneurysms. The characteristics of these aneurysms are as follows:

2.2. Prevalence and Incidence

Advancements in neuroimaging technology have driven recent interest in the epidemiology of unruptured intracranial aneurysms. Before the 1990s, published population-based studies were based on the incidence of hospital-admitted aneurysmal SAH, or of cerebral aneurysms detected on an overall autopsy or random autopsy basis of which between 9 and 51 cases out of 100,000 had SAH. Prevalence, utilizing cerebral angiography, largely centered on the prevalence of coarctation of the aorta, such as in the study using increased on the population-based prevalence in roentgenographic studies. Annual incidence rates of SAH were typically reported between six and 19 per 100,000 per year, and women were more frequently affected than men. Ärvelin-Forsel et al. and Longstreth et al. calculated the prevalence of unruptured intracranial aneurysms. In the latter study, the prevalence of computed tomographic angiography (CTA)-detected aneurysms greater than or equal to 7 mm was 7.5 percent based on a prevalence group. This number increased up to 10 percent when two additional cross-sectional studies were added with inclusion of a small number of persons evaluated with CTA.

Prevalence and incidence. Approximately 6 million people in the United States have an unruptured brain aneurysm, or one in 50 people. Larger aneurysms affect around 25,000 people annually in the United States. Aneurysms are more prevalent in women and are especially common in those aged 35–60. On a global scale, the prevalence of brain aneurysms is estimated based on Aneurysm Screening Study results.

3. Alcohol Consumption and Its Effects on the Brain

Long-term, chronic alcohol use can damage the brain in areas associated with memory, learning, emotion, and decision-making. Brain atrophy (wasting away); a decrease in the size of brain cells; a reduction in the metabolism of glucose, the brain's fuel; increased brain ventricle (cavities in the brain that hold cerebrospinal fluid); and damage to white matter can also occur. Ultimately, the results can lead to alcohol-related brain damage and a defect in thinking processing as well as a defect in your ability to sense time and location. Such effects, when used over extended periods, can be annoying and frustrating to long-term abusers.

Short-term effects of drinking might include: - Problems with balance, coordination, judgment, and emotion. - Poor motor coordination and vision, as well as slower and impaired reflexes. - Emotional, cognitive, and memory impairments, making it difficult to think clearly. - Sluggishness or drowsiness, eventually leading to unconsciousness and the possibility of death. - Potentially life-threatening alcohol poisoning symptoms.

Drinking alcohol in moderation is generally safe for most people if they are of legal drinking age and do so responsibly. When an individual overindulges or frequently consumes too much alcohol within a single session, it may impair brain function, which can lead to unsafe behaviors. Chronic, long-term alcohol use can change brain structure and impact memory, decision-making, and impulse control. Alcohol can also lead to addiction, or alcohol use disorder. Compared to other tissues within the body, the brain also has a higher susceptibility to alcohol-induced injury.

3.1. Short-Term Effects of Alcohol on the Brain

It can also lead to depression-like sluggishness and even the end of the brain, which is important for neural signaling and other physiological processes. Scientists have identified ethanol in alcoholic beverages, in large part, but these additional brain depressants are also to blame. Psychoactive agents that contain ethanol have the following: any beverage with 5% or more ethanol; a wine bottle (made from fermented grapes as well as other fruits) has the most ethanol at 9-16 percent per bottle. Mild euphoria, talkativeness, and even temporary memory loss are just a few short-term consequences of reduced excitation triggered by alcohol. Alcohol use also affects judgment, resulting in engaging in unswayed actions such as unprotected intercourse.

Huge numbers of American adults believe one of the best parts about coming in from the heat is enjoying an ice-cold adult beverage to make it even more enjoyable. But individuals should also be aware of the short-term effects of alcohol on the brain so they know when to put down the glass. When ingested, alcohol, which can contain 40% or greater concentration, is distributed through the tissues and fluids of the body, including the infamous blood-brain barrier. When it comes to short-term consequences, the sedative effect is the most commonly regarded alcohol-related action on the brain, which is also called reducing natural excitation. This reduction in physiological response is why a person gets wobbly, confused, and sleepy after having one too many drinks. Less excitation is the net

result, whether for the brain function or a muscular
activity.

3.2. Long-Term Effects of Alcohol on the Brain

Effect of regular drinking on the human brain: New research perspectives. Chronic alcoholism results in a variety of acute and chronic impacts on the human brain, ranging from occasional free radical changes and the development of hepatic encephalopathies to dyscirculation states. Recently, digital imaging techniques have helped modern research clarify the long-term effects of chronic alcohol consumption on the brain. Loss of gray brain mass has been shown to be linked to long-term use of alcohol, and brain injuries account for 13% of the total gray mass loss per decade of alcohol use. Additionally, white brain volume is also reduced. The states of abstinence and withdrawal have been linked to a greater decrease in brain mass. Chronic alcohol use also has the potential to cause permanent behavioral disorders, physical and mental illness, personality disorders, and a long-term increase in psychosocial problems. Brain mass shrinkage and white brain mass reduction in alcoholics is also caused by general brain mass shrinkage resulting from hepatic encephalopathies and brain electrolyte disorders caused by fluid clogging, as well as by associated cerebral atrophy or excessive vasculature clogging. Brain atrophy and white brain mass reduction as a result of aging are directly related to structural age-related changes in the brain, which can be corrected by calculating the generalized brain mass reduction due to inflammation, alcoholic brain mass reduction, and general brain mass reduction with aging in percentages. This is because the relative percentage lower factors of the three reduced values are also similar to the relative percentage factors of another, because the decline in the mass values of the alcoholic brain and the mass total collapse of the brain of age are directly related to estimator brain, white and intracranial matter. Additionally, the candidate's final brain survival is linked to hierarchical atrophy of the brain (evaluated using the same percentile relative percentage method) on the basis of further atrophy of the whole brain as a decline in the mass of white and intracranial brain. In the postnatal stage, atrophy of the brain leads to a collapse in overall brain size. Alcohol-induced permanent alterations to the brain that cause an aneurysm also include chronic growth of the muscular layers of the arteries and arterioles, which result in stiffer, less elastic cerebral arteries. Postsynthetrical wet brain weight increase was considerably higher in alcohol addicts who were middle-aged at death and very quickly began drinking.

4. The Relationship Between Alcohol Consumption and Brain Aneurysms

The reason for sudden ruptures of aneurysms is not firmly established, but certain demographic, genetic, and environmental factors have been determined. Several studies have shown that high-risk drugs, including alcohol and non-steroidal anti-inflammatory drugs, are linked to the development of aneurysms. Heavy alcohol use can cause stressful episodes everywhere and high blood pressure, especially in the submucosal blood vessels. Studies of data from the hospital database show that some SSRIs, which are widely used drugs to treat alcoholism, can also cause cerebral aneurysms. Heavy use is associated with excessive stress. In Great Britain, 90% of patients with alcohol-induced damage, such as aneurysms and intracranial aneurysms. Therefore, individuals with a history of heavy alcohol use should perform an MRI to control an aneurysm in the brain.

Is there a link between alcohol consumption and the occurrence of an aneurysm in the brain? This remains a hot topic. The research offers even antagonistic results. Aneurysm is a silent killer threatening thousands of people. It is difficult to diagnose, especially when 50% of all aneurysms coexist with sudden ruptures, leading to irreversible damage to the body. One of the most vulnerable areas of the body for this type of musculo-membranous disease is the human brain. Spontaneous bleeding in the brain leads to various symptoms, such as headaches, nausea, vomiting and in the worst case unconsciousness.

4.1. Studies and Research Findings

There is ongoing debate of how to define the most informative reference category and whether adjustment for potential confounders influences the association between alcohol consumption and cardiovascular risk. Finally, trials of drugs to increase alcohol consumption for the prevention of cardiovascular disease are monitored but are not currently in progress.

In addition, the time of drinking was ascertained for each alcoholic beverage. Overall, no significant differences were observed between cases and controls for alcohol consumption. The researchers suggested moderate consumption of alcohol to be associated with a decreased risk of intracranial aneurysm. Larger and better-designed clinical studies might show a different picture. The researchers proposed that these results should be hypothesis-generating rather than firm evidence for an anti-vascular effect of alcohol consumption. In addition, alcoholism can cause liver diseases which seem to predispose to intracranial aneurysms.

One large study reviewed patients' brain images and asked how often they drank alcohol. The study found that people who had at least one aneurysm were 50% more likely to be moderate drinkers. Research has suggested that some of the same behaviors that may increase the risk of a brain aneurysm, particularly smoking, may also raise the risk of having a stroke. On the other hand, many doctors say one or two drinks a day may help protect the heart and lower the risks of a heart attack, cardiac arrest, or a first stroke. If you have a brain aneurysm, it's important to talk to a doctor about the potential risks and benefits of some activities. Call 911 immediately if you experience any of the signs and symptoms of a brain aneurysm, such as a severe headache or loss of vision. A prospective study assessed the impact of alcohol consumption on aneurysmal subarachnoid hemorrhage. Patients were interviewed within three weeks of the onset of the hemorrhage using food frequency questionnaires with specific questions about alcoholic and non-alcoholic drinks, serving size, and frequency of drinking.

People have been studying alcohol's potential effects on brain aneurysms for several years. Some researchers have looked at medical records to compare patients with and without brain aneurysms, while others have asked patients about their alcohol and drug habits.

5. Risk Factors for Brain Aneurysms

About 10% of people who have an immediate family relative with a brain aneurysm will also have an aneurysm. So far, researchers have identified multiple helix-link peptide 2 on chromosome 1 as an important gene related to aneurysm formation and rupture. Having another condition such as polycystic kidney disease, Marfan syndrome, Ehlers-Danlos syndrome, and certain types of coarctation of the aorta can also increase the odds of having a brain aneurysm. People with a known hereditary predisposition to aneurysms, even if they don't have a diagnosed medical condition, should be vaccinated. Patients and people who are living with it on a daily basis in their families should know the signs and symptoms of a ruptured brain aneurysm in order to get help as soon as possible. Once a person gets diagnosed with a brain aneurysm, there are certain bad habits or living conditions that might potentially exacerbate an unfavorable disease process.

Various risk factors are associated with the development of a brain aneurysm, according to experts and scientists. Some of these factors are not within a patient's control, but some more lifestyle-related factors could potentially be addressed to help a person avoid developing a brain aneurysm. It's been estimated that around 2% of people in the population have a brain aneurysm, which is a weakened blood vessel bulge in one of their arteries. The more aneurysms a person has, the greater their risk of a significant rupture and bleed.

5.1. Genetic Factors

There are three specific genetic factors either singly or in combination that may predispose patients to a brain aneurysm: 1) vascular subtype; 2) size of the original brain aneurysm wall; and 3) the presence or absence of certain technical and physical changes that make the brain aneurysm more likely to leak. Atherosclerotic brain aneurysms are far more likely to be genetic in origin compared to other non-atherosclerotic brain aneurysms. Atherosclerotic brain aneurysms are part of a body-wide process, atherosclerosis, that may be genetic in nature. Simply based on feature size, an unruptured brain aneurysm that measures greater than or equal to seven millimeters has a 7.5 times greater risk of subsequent rupture compared to one that is smaller than seven millimeters (regardless of other factors).

Brain aneurysms can occur due to a variety of factors. While many instances occur randomly or by chance, genetics are known to play a role in increasing one's risk of developing brain aneurysms. Stress and alcohol consumption can both increase the risk of developing brain aneurysms because they can raise blood pressure. Ongoing high blood pressure can weaken the walls of the arteries, making developing brain aneurysms more likely. Hypertension is high blood pressure, and patients with hypertension have even higher odds of having a brain aneurysm.

5.2. Lifestyle Factors

Hypertension cannot only contribute to the formation of aneurysms by damaging the spiraled vascular wall in the brain but also increase the likelihood of their rupture. In addition, higher socioeconomic status, which can come with higher stress and/or societal factor-related risks, has been associated with an increased likelihood for having an unruptured brain aneurysm in more than one large study. A study from Japan also showed a 1.78-fold increased risk for the presence of an aneurysm in those with diabetes, adjusted for all the other aneurysm risk factors. These factors taken together underscore the importance of understanding the lifestyle habits an individual has in the assessment of brain aneurysm risk.

There are several modifiable risk factors, mostly related to lifestyle, that are thought to contribute to the formation and the rupture of an aneurysm in the brain. Cigarette smoking is the most researched lifestyle factor in this context, and the carbon monoxide and endothelial damage from smoking make aneurysms more prone to rupture. For example, a large longitudinal study from Japan reported a hazard ratio of 3.16 in those who smoked over 40 pack-years, which was higher than quitting smoking upon diagnosis (HR 2.14) or at least 3 years prior to the study (HR 2.46). Alcohol, specifically its use or abuse, is not thoroughly researched in the context of brain aneurysms. One study from Taiwan showed an independent inverse association (OR 0.64) between alcohol use and the occurrence of intracranial aneurysms, while the other studies haven't noted an association with aneurysm rupture.

6. Symptoms and Warning Signs of Brain Aneurysms

Identifying the potential signs and symptoms of brain aneurysms could make the difference between walking away without any residual deficit and dying or living with one or more visible or hidden deficits. An individual might experience a "sentinel" or "warning" leak and feel differently than he or she has in the past and not feel quite right, and can seek immediate medical attention. This simple effort can mean many extra years of life for an individual. In some ways, a deep-seated aneurysm will look like hemorrhagic stroke in terms of symptoms. If an aneurysm bursts, its symptoms can also include: a severe, sudden, and rumbly headache, often described as the "worst headache of my life"; neck stiffness; nausea; vomiting; sensitivity to light; confusion or sleepiness; and new or worse headache. It is very common for these symptoms to occur so quickly that they are not immediately explainable. In fact, most aneurysms do not have symptoms until an individual has a serious event, such as a stroke.

When a brain aneurysm occurs, the weakened blood vessel becomes vulnerable to ballooning outwards, with or without bursting. The warning signs of a brain aneurysm are typically known as "sentinel" headaches or "warning" leaks. Two-thirds of patients only experience a single or more of these symptoms, and therefore recognizing the signs and getting attention straight away could help save your life. Clinical care for a brain aneurysm could vary between patients and can affect the necessary treatments.

7. Diagnosis and Treatment Options for Brain Aneurysms

One possible treatment is clipping, which involves a neurosurgeon removing a portion of the skull to reach the aneurysm. The surgeon then employs a gold clip to limit blood flow to the weakened portion of the artery. Another treatment involves filling the aneurysm with different coil materials to initiate blood clot formation that will stop the blood from flowing to the aneurysm altogether. Endovascular coiling is a less invasive approach than clipping and may come with fewer risks, especially for patients in poorer health. When a ruptured brain aneurysm is identified and diagnosed as the cause of the bleeding, nimodipine, which prevents and reduces vasospasms, is administered. This drug can help prevent delayed vasospasms and help improve neurologic outcomes, but it contains some toxic elements as well. High blood pressure can be treated with various drugs and can be placed in a position of deformation to reduce the blood flow to the portion of the brain thus affected.

If you are experiencing any of these symptoms or suspect that you have a brain aneurysm, the first step should be to see a doctor. There are various diagnostic procedures that work together to provide an accurate overview of the aneurysm for doctors to create a comprehensive treatment plan. Depending on the patient's symptoms and condition, these tests can include a lumbar puncture or CT scan. However, occasionally a CT angiogram, digital subtraction angiography (DSA), or magnetic resonance angiography (MRA) may be necessary as well. There is no universal treatment for every case of brain aneurysm. Many factors can influence which treatments will be successful for you, including your age and other conditions.

8. Prevention Strategies for Brain Aneurysms

Adopting particular lifestyle habits like a healthy diet that helps maintain control over low high blood pressure, stop addiction and abuse, and using practices that are not involved in the development of viral and bacterial infective aneurysms is part of the preventive approach to stroke. Similarly, prophylactic coiling or other endovascular therapy, followed by magnetic resonance, are further prevention methods in a person at an identification. "Against more than 7,000 individuals, the Yessenian did not have a single inpatient producing medical problems linked to the coil wear-offs. We achieved 98 per cent of the segmental occlusions at the Aneurysms," he said. If you would like to discuss this option individually, contact the office of your primary adult or dial 410-12213.

There is no way to completely prevent a brain aneurysm from developing, but making lifestyle changes and seeking necessary medical treatments are two important prevention strategies. Some individuals may be born with a reduced number of connective tissue elements in the walls of arterial blood vessels in the brain. Yet, not all modifications to the brain pathological condition are efficient in avoiding an aneurysm, if a person worries that one could be developing. By addressing certain aspects of an at-risk patient's life, how long they exist, and the diseases they have developed, functional prevention measures and preventive programmes that make it possible to refuse to occur are part of this plan.

8.1. Lifestyle Changes

Get moving. Engaging in daily exercise for 30 minutes on all days of the week is one of the easiest ways to lower your likelihood of brain aneurysm. Aim for 150 minutes of physical activity per week, or 20 to 25 minutes of exercise per day. Changing your exercises, as well as doing moderate-intensity cardio and bodyweight workouts, can help you avoid burnout and stay motivated to maintain a daily routine. Sudden physical exertion, such as grunting while lifting a heavy object, may increase the risk of subarachnoid hemorrhage (a certain type of stroke caused by a ruptured brain aneurysm). Easing your way into more rigorous exercise, such as jogging and strength training, and ensuring that your body is warm and well-stretched will help minimize this danger. Subarachnoid hemorrhage can be aggravated by high blood pressure and cardiovascular failure. To avoid potential health concerns, such as rupturing an undiagnosed aneurysm, seek guidance from your healthcare provider before starting a new workout regimen.

Say no to alcohol and illegal narcotics. Alcohol use is a known risk factor, and cocaine can cause the rupture of an aneurysm, doctors said. Make a consultation with your healthcare provider or a certified addiction specialist for assistance diverting from compulsive drug and alcohol usage.

Quit smoking. Each puff of tobacco is a known threat factor for both brain aneurysms and a number of other lethal and chronic health conditions. You are likely to suffer from high blood pressure, as smoking impedes the circulation of oxygen to the vein. Cerebral atherosclerosis is another threat connected with smoking. Schedule a consultation with your healthcare provider in order to utilize tools like quit smoking aids and personalized behavioral change methods to tackle this bad habit.

Eat healthier. The DASH (Dietary Approaches to Stop Hypertension) diet, which emphasizes fruits, vegetables, whole grains, and low-fat dairy, may help lower your risk of hypertension and atherosclerosis. Keep your blood sugar monitored. Exercising regularly and avoiding high-sodium, high-fat, and overly processed foods will help you achieve this.

Your lifestyle can influence the risk of a variety of conditions, including brain aneurysms. These are some of the things you can do to lower your risk:

8.2. Medical Interventions

One of these studies found that 2.7% of patients with specialized disease (similar to ADPKD in that there are many small kidney cysts present) exhibited intracranial aneurysms, and aneurysms were found in three of these patients. The goal of medicine is to increase the chances of successful renal transplantation in ADPKD sufferers. The presence of an aneurysm is a contraindication to transplantation unless the aneurysm has been treated. This is especially true for those who have had a stroke or have uncontrolled high blood pressure. The following is a summary of the treatment options available:

Medical interventions. Medical interventions, if used to prevent the development of aneurysms, theoretically could affect the progression of ADPKD in the form of aneurysms, although no trials are currently available to determine the value of these interventions. The primary medical goal in reducing a patient's risk of a future SAH is the maintenance of normal blood pressure to prevent vessels from undergoing the vasospasms that may cause an aneurysmal rupture. Although no preventative methods are currently known, several studies have determined risk factors that may increase the chance of aneurysms by weakening the blood vessel walls. Based on these findings, we believe it would be helpful for patients with a confirmed family history of aneurysms to seek advice on the prevention and treatment of these conditions. These studies provide evidence of the predisposition toward aneurysms, an unusual creation of an aneurysm from a smaller arterial vessel that has not developed with age or when hypertension is present.

9. Conclusion and Future Directions

The aims of the current review were as follows: to explore the association between alcoholism and brain aneurysms. The animal studies involving aneurysms were also checked and included. Recommendations for the surgeons to treat the aneurysm based on the alcoholism treatment were also covered. The first brain aneurysm clip reported by Dandy in 1937 due to alcohol-induced disappearance of the wall. But he didn't mention the mechanism of the wall dissection. According to the studies, alcohol hinders aneurysmal neck healing. Future studies are required to determine the benefit of treatment in patients after brain aneurysm rupture. It is also necessary to investigate the change in the protein level due to alcohol. In the future, we plan to calculate the average diameter of all arteries including the brain artery. In addition, we would like to investigate MST1, cell, and fibrous expression patterns for autophagy.

This review includes both animal and human studies to cover all aspects that support the relationship between alcohol and the risk of brain aneurysms. Alcoholic arteritis causes damage to the kidney, pancreas, nerve cells, heart muscles, and smooth muscles, and damages the blood vessels. Alcohol is clearly a potential compound that causes degeneration of the arterial wall and development of berry aneurysms, and may be a potential cause of new bleeds from ruptured aneurysms. This retrogressive part that also extends to the parent artery is the reason to simplify the treatment of the aneurysm during the acute phase.

The Relationship Between Alcohol Consumption and Brain Aneurysms

1. Introduction to Brain Aneurysms and Alcohol Consumption

Alcohol is known to be a contributing factor in 10% of non-traumatic subarachnoid hemorrhages - bleeding associated with ruptured aneurysms. Some reports have also found that among people who have a primary subarachnoid hemorrhage that is not associated with head trauma, 18.5% might be heavy alcohol users. At the same time, a few studies have looked at the relationship between alcohol consumption and subarachnoid hemorrhage incidence. Some researchers have questioned whether alcohol might not be a factor in causing aneurysm formation and subsequent rupture. Others have looked at the relationship between alcohol use and the risk of aneurysm enlargement in people who have not had rupture.

A brain aneurysm (also commonly called a cerebral aneurysm or a brain or cerebral aneurysm) is an abnormal swelling or bulge in the wall of a brain artery. A rarer form of aneurysm is when it is not associated with a widening (or ballooning), but it creates a small blister-like outpouching from the side wall of an artery (like a bubble on a tire). Aneurysms typically develop at the point where a blood vessel diverts from the main artery, which is called a bifurcation point, or at a "T" branch site, which is called a trifurcation site. The larger aneurysms that develop a "Y" shaped formation at the branching site are called multilobed aneurysms. Aneurysms, like varicose veins, are areas where the artery wall is weaker and are more blood dilated. Smoking is the leading risk factor for causing aneurysm enlargement and rupture.

2. Understanding the Mechanisms of Brain Aneurysm Formation

Aneurysms are uncontrolled and localized dilations of arteries. To date, the underlying mechanisms are not fully elucidated. However, it is clear that aneurysm formation is complex and requires the cooperation of various cell types and chemical messengers, such as metalloproteases. An incomplete, but not exclusive, list of the different regulatory mechanisms includes inflammation, cytokines, proteases, growth factors, and vascular smooth cells. In principle, there are two different types of aneurysms: saccular and fusiform; they can also appear as mixed forms.

Aneurysms are uncontrolled and localized dilations that can affect any artery in the human body. These formations are dangerous because they bear a higher risk of leaking and/or rupturing. Although they can appear in any part of the body, intracranial aneurysms are considerably dangerous and are often subjects of study. In the cerebral vasculature, these structures develop from the basal arteries. The severe hemorrhage that a ruptured aneurysm can cause is associated with high mortality and severe morbidity. Thus, prognosis is poor. Despite the technological progression over the past decades, invasive and non-invasive secondary prevention still face a significant proportion of morbidity and mortality. A better understanding of the mechanisms involved in the formation of brain aneurysms would improve prevention.

In this issue of Hypertension, Xiang et al show in a canine aneurysm model that alcohol can increase wall inflammation and MMP-2 activity in the cerebrovascular structure downstream of the aneurysm. This partially explains increases in urealy iron mechanisms and scar formation and thrombus organization in the ILT.

3. Effects of Alcohol on Blood Vessels and Aneurysm Development

So, can it therefore be concluded that any change in blood vessel function (due to excessive alcohol consumption) can increase the risk of aneurysm development? It would seem a fair hypothesis, although a direct connection between alcohol and aneurysms is yet to be made. This article aims to evaluate this relationship, starting with the effects of alcohol on blood vessels before discussing other, more general potential risk factors. Vascular smooth muscle cells are the primary component of arteries and arterioles and are responsible for a variety of neurological, endocrine, and vasocrine functions. They're also responsible for minimizing shear stress by controlling blood flow.

The effects of alcohol on various bodily organs and systems are myriad, from changes in the heart to the risk of such conditions as obesity, diabetes, and dementia. Alcohol can also have devastating effects on blood vessels, which will be looked at in more detail. Blood vessels are responsible for the transportation of blood around the body, bringing oxygen and nutrients to tissues such as the heart and brain. In terms of brain health, vascular function is clearly incredibly important. To be more specific, it has been noted that the arterial wall in the brain is directly susceptible to changes in blood pressure, which can lead to the formation of aneurysms. An aneurysm is effectively a weakness in a blood vessel that leads to a bulge. If this bulge bursts, it can lead to a bleed on the brain called a subarachnoid haemorrhage, which is associated with an extremely high fatality rate.

4. Alcohol-Induced Hypertension and Its Impact on Aneurysm Risk

Gender variations in some of the evidence culled from these studies point to a heightened susceptibility to intracranial aneurysm rupture due to smoking and heavy drinking in both sexes. Genetic nuances in alcohol breakdown and greater sensitivity of the female brain to alcohol's detrimental consequences are likewise crucial to future alcohol and aneurysm research. Effects of alcohol consumption on those factors that can predict the growth and rupture of a cerebral aneurysm will likewise need to be investigated. More research is also called for on the protective and detrimental actions of alcohol in lab animals with induced aneurysms representing both common and rare types of aneurysm.

As an independent risk factor for stroke and other cerebrovascular pathologies, high blood pressure is intricately associated with the formation, enlargement, and rupture of intracranial aneurysms. An aneurysm is characterized as a bulge in one of the blood vessels within the brain, and it may continue to expand until it ruptures, causing bleeding that may be dangerous, disabling, or even fatal. Alcohol abuse and even moderate drinking are both associated with greater blood pressure readings. According to some research, the connection between alcohol consumption and hypertension is more pronounced in men than women, which is noteworthy in light of certain interesting results of research into gender-specific predictors for intracranial aneurysm growth and rupture. Evidence also suggests that frequent heavy episodic drinking, which is defined as four or more alcoholic beverages consumed on one occasion, is associated with a several-day rise in blood pressure, which may add to regularly high blood pressure readings.

5. Role of Inflammation and Oxidative Stress in Aneurysm Formation

Oxidative stress is defined as 'an imbalance between oxidants and antioxidants in favor of the oxidants, leading to a disruption of redox signaling and control and/or molecular damage'. In oxidative stress, the overproduction of reactive nitrogen species (RNS) and reactive oxygen species (ROS) is involved. As a biochemical reaction, oxidative stress is created when O2 oxidation products, superoxide radical anion O2-, and hydrogen peroxide are created. These radicals and derivatives have the ability to act as secondary messengers in small amounts. Oxidative stress occurs at higher doses of superoxide radical anion, where the target cells are overloaded with oxidants, and the intracellular redox balance is disturbed. The change of redox in cells can provoke downstream cell stress, which further induces a pro-inflammatory response. In addition, oxidative stress can also induce cellular damage and thus initiate the development of IA.

The formation of brain aneurysms is a complex process, and inflammation and oxidative stress are both thought to be involved. Inflammation is a host-defense mechanism, and when inflammation is activated, it is involved in tissue repair. However, if the inflammation cannot be resolved, the host becomes injured. Chronic inflammation is one trigger for the destruction of organ function and the onset of a range of diseases. The internal aspects of inflammation on the circulatory system consist of atherosclerosis, on artery walls, and aneurysms. An intracranial aneurysm is a blood-filled dilation of an artery in the brain. As they can burst spontaneously and become life-threatening, the relationship between aneurysms and chronic inflammation needs to be formally validated.

6. Genetic Factors and Alcohol-Related Aneurysm Susceptibility

Additionally, alcohol may have changed vasodilator substance production or influenced the shape and diameter of arteries, raising blood pressure and causing a localized area of wall weakness. A study conducted on Finnish individuals emphasizes the potential role of heredity in the relationship between alcohol and aneurysm occurrence. In fact, the authors argue that Finnish citizens have an inherited predisposition to aneurysm formation that causes them to form more cysts as a result of aneurysm. This genetic weakness (incompletely penetrable) exacerbates aneurysm formation but must be coupled with certain environmental features, such as specific nutritional factors that favor cyst formation, for the first vessel injury that induces aneurysm.

Nowadays, the study of the relationship between genetic factors and sporadic brain aneurysms focuses on the possibility of identifying genes that may cause a predisposition to the disease. As a result, aneurysms probably occur as the final consequence of a complex interaction between multiple genetic and environmental factors. Ethanol can have a vast array of effects on human health, both damaging and beneficial, based on the level of exposure. At low doses, alcohol may have some advantageous properties, such as altering cell membranes and fluidity, stabilizing cell membranes, and reducing intracerebral edema. It has been suggested that alcoholic individuals may also have altered cerebral vasculature, resulting in the loosening of connections between endothelial cells.

7. Clinical Studies and Epidemiological Evidence

Evidence acquisition was undertaken to locate all pertinent research across five significant electronic databases, using a combination of medical subject headings and text keywords in the search. The total of the research works were found throughout the query. Eight cohort investigation studies were identified, followed by the originating data being reviewed by two of the authors. A total of 149,645 research participants contributed to the case analyses. Data from these studies suggest that the role of alcohol as a possible risk factor in the development of new aneurysms in the brain is complex. Population-based data is distributed in this domain, with no definitive conclusions. Longitudinal, case-controlled research efforts are required so that the relationships between the cerebral aneurysms and alcohol could be researched in the future.

In order to circumvent potential harmful effects resulting from untreated ruptured aneurysms, being knowledgeable about people who are at heightened risk for de novo aneurysm formation is of high clinical significance. In light of the fact that some cohort research studies have identified excessive alcohol consumption as a risk factor for developing a new brain aneurysm, that's why we are attempting to search for potential relationships between the brain aneurysms and alcohol consumption.

8. Symptoms and Diagnosis of Brain Aneurysms

The development of intracranial hypertension can be accompanied by attacks of tinnitus, hearing loss, and periodic violation of the functions of the optic nerve, eye muscles, and trigeminal nerve. The main methods of instrumental examination for the diagnosis of aneurysms are: computed tomography (CT) and magnetic resonance imaging (MRI) of the brain, sagittal angiography and its modifications (transosseous angiography, contrast-CT and MRI), and three-dimensional angiography (3D regression), which allows to obtain a wide cross-section before performed surgery.

Aneurysm (dilatation and tortuosity of a vessel) can have a variety of clinical manifestations, but most often the disease occurs asymptomatically. In the acute development of the process, the clinical picture is urgent and life-threatening, accompanied by severe chronic. It has a headache, dizziness, vomiting, signs of meningeal syndrome, paresis of cranial nerves, and characterizes disturbance of consciousness. Inspection of the optic fundus reveals increased organ tone and slightly blurry eye ground vessels, the development of single or multiple hemorrhages with a diameter of 0.1-0.5 mm. At the beginning of the inflow, hemorrhages are usually flame-shaped and single, mainly on one half of the eye ground, located on the border of the central and medium or middle and peripheral zones from the temporal side to the optic disc. With the increasing frequency of hemorrhages and their accumulation, larger zones of lesions appear that grow.

9. Treatment Options and Management Strategies

Treatment for a brain aneurysm ranges from watchful waiting to endovascular coiling or neurosurgical clipping. Both employ techniques in which metal, either in the form of a coil or clip, is used to isolate the aneurysm from the circulation. The choice of treatment modality should be individualized to the unique patient, aneurysm, and location. The size and shape of the aneurysm, the patient's age and general health, history of brain hemorrhage or multiple aneurysms, and other risk factors for aneurysm bleeding such as smoking or high blood pressure, influence the recommendation for intervention. Patients may wish to get a second opinion and consider more conservative treatment options while weighing risks and benefits of invasive procedures. In this review, we discuss endovascular coiling, neurosurgical methods, bypass techniques, and exploratory treatments such as parent vessel occlusion.

Early animal studies and limited human studies suggested that alcohol might promote brain aneurysm formation. More recently, the findings have been somewhat mixed regarding the relationship between brain aneurysms and drinking alcohol. One large study published last year showed no increase in the risk of aneurysms from heavy drinking. It seems, however, that a history of heavy drinking might increase the risk of aneurysm rupture for certain smaller aneurysms in both smokers and some types of non-smokers. These results could be consistent with an alcohol-related stress on smaller aneurysms that causes them to weaken and rupture. It is not clear what effect, if any, light to moderate drinking has on aneurysms. Heavy drinking might also increase the risk of hypertension and liver disease, which in turn could raise the risk of aneurysms, albeit indirectly.

10. Prevention and Lifestyle Modifications

If you have a family history of brain aneurysms, there are other potential preventive strategies that you can change or modify in your lifestyle, such as high blood pressure, cigarette smoking, heavy alcohol consumption, drug abuse, stress, and thyroid abnormalities. These risk factors will also help reduce the risk of developing a brain aneurysm. Research has found that natural elements (like flavonoids, a substance in blueberries), fat, and calorie content have very significant results in the development of brain aneurysms. In knowledge, research shows that individuals who have three or four servings of fruit have a 37% lower risk of a brain aneurysm.

The initial measure to prevent a brain aneurysm is by avoiding the causative factors. Alcohol and tobacco are known to be significant risk factors for developing a brain aneurysm. By making lifestyle adjustments and changing individual behavior, this can contribute much to preventing an aneurysm. If you consume alcohol often, then slowly lessen your alcohol consumption. Or, you can find alternate things that can give you relaxation, such as hobbies and some fun activities. You can also find emotional support from your family and friends related to stress handling and can also join some stress-related clubs. Aneurysms can naturally occur over time and with age. Injury will also increase the risk of an aneurysm. About 80% of patients with subarachnoid hemorrhage from a ruptured aneurysm have high blood pressure. High blood pressure produces additional stress on the arterial walls and the force of blood flow. The pressure can increase the size of an aneurysm and also increase the risk of rupture. Many young people suffer from this type of medical illness due to drug abuse like cocaine and accidents. They widely suffer from an aneurysm with alcohol consumption. It's possible to already have aneurysms and risk bleeding in the brain without even knowing. Maintaining preventative lifestyle changes and seeking medical care can help reduce the risk of bleeding from untreated aneurysms.

11. Public Health Implications and Awareness Campaigns

Conclusions: It is not yet possible to state to a high level of confidence that alcohol consumption is a risk factor for brain aneurysms. However, available epidemiological data, some using valid instruments, and most accounting for comorbidities, are suggestive of its role in the development of aneurysms. Therefore, definitive conclusions await further epidemiological investigation, utilizing large sample sizes and accounting for known aneurysm risk factors. Solely PSA programs and increased aneurysm education will most likely only have a minimal impact on reducing aneurysm incidence and rupture unless tailored therapeutic and preventive measures are also incorporated. Given the societal impact incurred by brain aneurysms at the individual and family levels as well as by public healthcare systems, more research to identify and validate risk factors and potential targets is warranted to prevent these common and deadly conditions. Strong evidence already supports the lifesaving potential of a polypathology approach for SAH prevention.

The implications and consequences of an aneurysm range from personal tragedy on the individual and the family level to broader societal ripples. The healthcare system bears enormous costs associated with physical and rehabilitative care for survivors of aneurysm ruptures. In addition, a disproportionate percentage of those who suffer a brain aneurysm are in the prime of their adult, productive lives when the event occurs. Furthermore, the majority of victims are women and, accordingly, the principal caretakers in most families. Consequently, in both the short and long run, a high personal, social, and fiscal burden accompanies the presence of unruptured aneurysms and SAH. Given the high percentage of individuals who die immediately or shortly after the rupture of an aneurysm (and never seek medical care or receive any diagnosis of their condition), the public is, at present, largely uninformed about the potential risks associated with an aneurysm diagnosis. Thus, from a preventive health standpoint, an education and awareness campaign seems wise, perhaps a "universal plan" to encourage imaging for anyone who wants it, combined with an educational component. Furthermore, there is currently a critical unmet need to educate the public on brain aneurysms and advocate for improved research and healthcare resources to address their early detection, prevention, and ultimately eradication.

12. Conclusion and Future Research Directions

Our current data presented here are from the first 100 patients enrolled and the first assessment point of heavy drinking, and we will continue to assess risks of aneurysm growth/rupture over time as this study continues. In conclusion, those who abused alcohol, but are now abstinent, have brain aneurysm growth/rupture rates that do not differ from rates among those who have never abused alcohol. Given the "dose-dependent" risk associated with heavy drinking (e.g., 6-10 drinks/day, 4-5 days/week for ≥ 1 yr, and 11 or more drinks in a day for only 1 report), irrespective of lifetime, factors that may precede brain aneurysm formation and assess the question of a direct effect of alcohol abuse on the formation of brain aneurysms are especially critical, as is continued research to investigate possible links between alcohol and increased risk for brain aneurysm growth/rupture or rebleeding of the aneurysm.

In summary, one pathway through which alcohol may lead to growth/rupture of brain aneurysms is by increasing blood pressure. Other predisposing factors for brain aneurysm growth or rupture include female gender, prior subarachnoid hemorrhage from another aneurysm, size of the aneurysm, history of smoking, presence of multiple aneurysms, and age. Whether your aneurysm was treated or not, and if treated, what kind of treatment you underwent, and how long ago a treatment was performed can also be important factors. Our study is the first to report on the history of heavy alcohol consumption as a risk factor for the future growth and/or rupture of unruptured brain aneurysms in patients followed over time regardless of the treatment status of their aneurysms. Although additional confirmatory research is necessary, once studied, treatments to prevent future aneurysm growth/rupture in patients who continue to drink heavily may differ from medical or surgical treatments to prevent growth/rupture for those who do not drink heavily.